American College of Physicians

HOME MEDICAL GUIDE *to*

BREAST
PROBLEMS

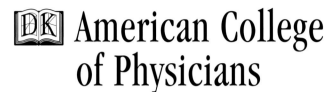 American College
of Physicians

HOME MEDICAL GUIDE *to*

BREAST
PROBLEMS

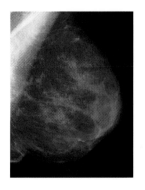

MEDICAL EDITOR
DAVID R. GOLDMANN, MD
ASSOCIATE MEDICAL EDITOR
DAVID A. HOROWITZ, MD

A DORLING KINDERSLEY BOOK

IMPORTANT

The American College of Physicians (ACP) Home Medical Guides provide general information on a wide range of health and medical topics. These books are not substitutes for medical diagnosis, and you should always consult your doctor on personal health matters before undertaking any program of therapy or treatment. Various medical organizations have different guidelines for diagnosis and treatment of the same conditions; the American College of Physician–American Society of Internal Medicine (ACP–ASIM) has tried to present a reasonable consensus of these opinions.

Material in this book was reviewed by the ACP–ASIM for general medical accuracy and applicability in the United States; however, the information provided herein does not necessarily reflect the specific recommendations or opinions of the ACP–ASIM. The naming of any organization, product, or alternative therapy in these books is not an ACP–ASIM endorsement, and the omission of any such name does not indicate ACP–ASIM disapproval.

DORLING KINDERSLEY

LONDON, NEW YORK, AUCKLAND, DELHI, JOHANNESBURG, MUNICH, PARIS, AND SYDNEY

DK www.dk.com

Senior Editors Jill Hamilton, Nicki Lampon

Senior Designer Jan English

DTP Design Jason Little

Editor Judit Z. Bodnar

Medical Consultant Kevin R. Fox, MD

Senior Managing Editor Martyn Page

Senior Managing Art Editor Bryn Walls

Published in the United States in 2000 by
Dorling Kindersley Publishing, Inc.
95 Madison Avenue, New York, New York 10016

2 4 6 8 10 9 7 5 3 1

Library of Congress Catalog Card Number 99-76863
ISBN 0-7894-4174-8

Reproduced by Colourscan, Singapore
Printed and bound in the United States by Quebecor World, Taunton, Massachusetts

3 8522 10045 5095

Contents

Know your breasts

In the developing fetus, the breasts start to develop very soon after conception and, to begin with, do so in the same way whether the baby is a boy or a girl.

DEVELOPING AND CHANGING

Five or six weeks after a baby is conceived, and while it is still only inches long, two ridges of tissue can be seen running from what will subsequently be the armpit to the groin. These ridges are called the "milk lines."

About six months into the pregnancy, special cells grow inward from the baby's nipples, and channels, or ducts, are formed. By the time the baby is born, the breast anatomy is in place in basic form. Some newborns have swollen or inflamed breasts from hormones passed to them through the placenta from their mother.

Most girls' breasts begin to develop between the ages of nine and eleven, but the process can begin earlier or later. Even when the breasts are fully grown, they are not capable of producing milk at this stage. It is not unusual for boys to experience some breast development during puberty as well, but this is only temporary and usually disappears within a year or two.

During pregnancy, a woman's breasts become much bigger and may double their weight as milk-producing

THE CHANGING BREAST
The breast structure of a lactating woman changes in response to hormones released during pregnancy. The nipples enlarge and darken, the milk-duct system expands, and more lobules are formed.

7

How the Breasts Develop

Breast development in females begins around the age of 9–11 years, although it may be earlier or later. The ovaries produce estrogen, leading to an accumulation of fat in the connective tissue and causing the breasts to enlarge.

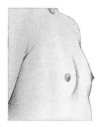

BEFORE PUBERTY THE
BREASTS ARE FLAT

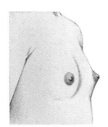

AREOLAE DEVELOP
AS BUDS

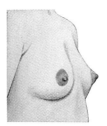

BREAST TISSUE AND
GLANDS GROW

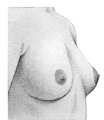

AREOLAE FLATTEN
OVER BREAST TISSUE

cells multiply and the system of ducts expands. The nipples turn darker, and blood vessels become more prominent. All these changes take place in response to various hormones that a woman produces while she is pregnant, and most are temporary. However, once the nipples have become darker, they stay that way because they contain more pigment than previously.

As we age, all our body tissues begin to lose their elasticity, and the breasts are no exception. They start to sag and, after menopause, become smaller because the decrease in levels of the female hormone estrogen causes the glands inside the breasts to shrink.

INSIDE THE BREAST

The easiest way to understand how the inside of the breast is formed is by comparing it to an upturned bush. Its "leaves" are known as lobules. They produce milk

The Anatomy of the Breasts

The breasts lie outside the ribcage and the pectoral muscles. They contain milk-secreting alveoli, and lacteal ducts carry the milk to the nipples. A network of lymph vessels and lymph nodes surrounding the breasts forms part of the immune system.

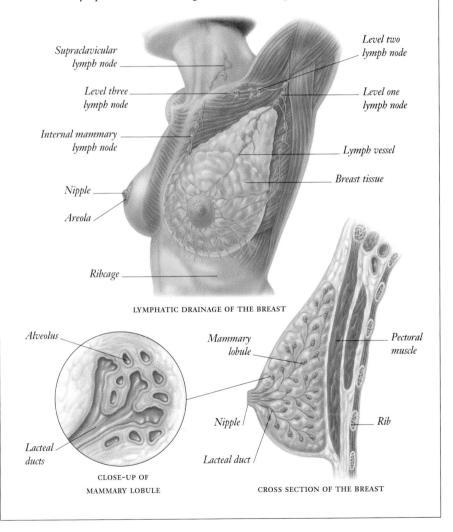

LYMPHATIC DRAINAGE OF THE BREAST

CLOSE-UP OF
MAMMARY LOBULE

CROSS SECTION OF THE BREAST

9

that drains along a network of small ducts through the "branches." These in turn drain into 12 or 15 major or large ducts that then empty onto the surface of the nipple. The nipple is the equivalent of the bush's trunk. As with a bush, the breast's branching network of ducts is irregular, not arranged symmetrically like the segments of an orange.

The spaces you would see between the leaves and the branches of a bush are filled inside the breast with connective tissue that provides structural support to the lobules and ducts. Around all of this is a layer of fat between the milk-producing parts of the breast and the skin. The breasts are supported by the chest muscles beneath them. Toning up these muscles with the right kind of exercise is the only way, apart from surgery, to change your appearance. Exercise does not have any effect on the size or shape of the breast tissue itself.

BREAST AWARENESS

Women used to be advised to examine their breasts carefully and regularly each month at the same point in their menstrual cycle. Not surprisingly, doing this made some women feel anxious. Others felt guilty if they failed to do it, and they felt somehow responsible if they later developed a problem.

Today, most doctors agree that the most important thing is "breast awareness" – knowing your own breasts so that you spot any unexpected change in them and can seek advice as soon as possible. What it means in practice is being thoroughly familiar with the appearance and texture of your breasts.

First, you should know what your breasts look like. It sounds obvious, but it is a good idea to get into the

Taking Care of Your Breasts

Personal awareness and routine screening are key to the early detection of possible breast problems. They may prompt more detailed examination of the breasts and early treatment for any disorder.

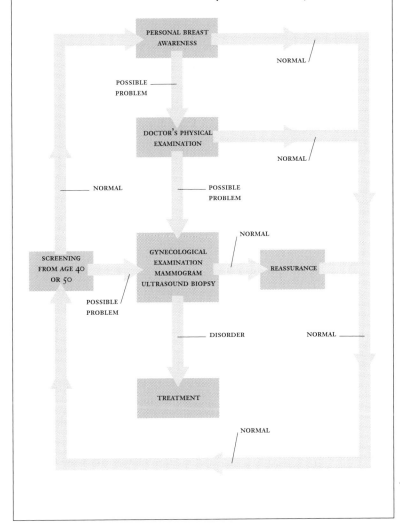

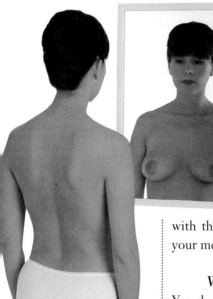

MIRROR INSPECTION
A basic awareness of how your breasts look in the mirror forms a good basis for detecting any general changes in their shape or skin texture.

habit of looking at your bare breasts in the mirror from time to time. Notice how they move as you hold your arms in various positions, so that you know what is normal for you. What you are looking for is a change in the shape of the breast, such as a dimpling of the skin, visible swelling of the breast, or a change in the nipple, such as "inversion" of the nipple.

You also need to know how your breasts feel. No one could be expected to find a lump when feeling her breast for the first time. You need experience before you can judge what is normal for you. Most women's breasts are a bit lumpy, especially in the days before a menstrual period is due. After their period, this lumpiness becomes less obvious or may disappear altogether. Start by feeling your breasts every day for a few days until you are familiar with their texture and know how it changes through your menstrual cycle.

WHAT IF YOU FIND A PROBLEM?

You should see your doctor right away if you notice any unusual change in your breasts, whether it is in the texture, the skin, or the nipple. Remember that roughly nine out of ten breast lumps are NOT cancerous.

Even if you do turn out to have a serious problem, there is absolutely no doubt that early diagnosis and treatment greatly increase the chances that the cancer or other disease will be cured completely.

KEY POINTS

- Be aware of the shape and feel of your breasts.
- Tell your doctor about any lumps or changes in the shape of your breasts.
- Nine out of ten breast lumps are not cancerous.

Breast screening

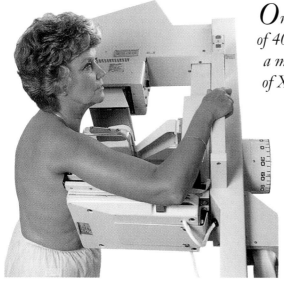

Once a woman reaches the age of 40, she will be advised to have a mammogram, a special kind of X-ray used to image breasts, once every year or two.

The aim of mammography is to detect breast cancer while it is still small and before it has spread in the breast or to other parts of the body.

There are a number of reasons why women are not normally screened before the age of 40:

HAVING A MAMMOGRAM
During a mammogram, each breast is placed on a photographic plate and gently compressed. This flattens the breast so that X-rays may be taken of as much breast tissue as possible.

- Breast cancer is less common in younger women.
- Mammography is less likely to detect abnormalities in women under the age of 40 because their breast tissue is denser than that of older women.
- There is no evidence that screening women before they reach 40 is cost-effective.

However, screening is recommended for any woman who is thought to be at particularly high risk of developing breast cancer (see pp.54–58). Studies are being done to evaluate whether another type of scan, magnetic resonance imaging (MRI), is useful in screening young women with a high risk for developing breast cancer. In general, however, screening with regular mammography is most effective in preventing death from breast cancer in women over the age of 50. The American Cancer Society recommends that women begin annual mammography screening at the age of 40. The guidelines used by various other medical organizations differ; for example, the National Cancer Institute suggests that women be screened every one to two years from age 40, while the American College of Physicians–American Society of Internal Medicine recommends screening every one or two years between the ages of 50 and 75.

MAMMOGRAPHY

You will be asked to undress to the waist and stand in front of the X-ray machine. The radiographer will position each breast in turn between two photographic plates so that it is compressed and flattened. A brief pulse of X-rays is then used to take images of each breast, normally two per breast on each visit. Some women find the experience uncomfortable, and a few say that it is painful, but for the majority there is no more than minor discomfort. In any case, it is all over very quickly.

The X-ray film is examined, and you will be told the results within a few days. A few women are asked to return for a second mammogram, sometimes because something has shown up and needs further investigation, or possibly due to technical difficulties with the original X-ray. Being called back may not mean a diagnosis of cancer. The medical staff will explain why the further check is needed.

MAMMOGRAM
This color-enhanced mammogram shows a normal breast in a woman of menopausal age.

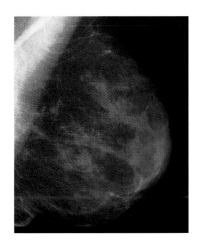

15

LITTLE CAUSE FOR ANXIETY

Although most women are reasonably relaxed about having a routine mammogram, being asked to return for a repeat test or further investigation is more likely to make you anxious.

Being anxious is natural enough, but the prospect may be less intimidating if you know that it is still unlikely that you will be found to have a serious problem.

The graph on the opposite page indicates that, for every 10,000 women who are examined using breast X-rays, only about 55 of them are found to have cancer, and their chances of successful treatment are greatly improved because the cancer has been detected at a relatively early stage.

INTERPRETING THE RESULTS
An experienced radiologist will scrutinize mammograms for any sign of abnormality.

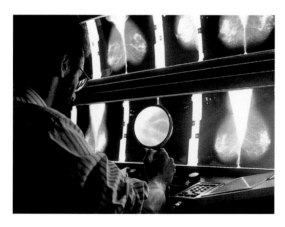

MAMMOGRAPHY – THE PROS AND CONS

● **Just having the test makes you anxious** True, but the exam itself does not last long, and, for the vast majority of women whose results are normal, the relief makes the temporary anxiety worthwhile.

● **What if a tumor is missed?** It is uncommon for a tumor not to be detected by mammography in women over 40.

● **A positive result is alarming and means you will need more tests** In about 50 in 1,000 women who are screened, an abnormality is found, but, after further investigation, the problem turns out not to be cancer.

Mammography

Of every 10,000 women who are given a mammogram, 500 will be recalled for assessment; 100 of these will have a surgical biopsy, and 55 will have cancers.

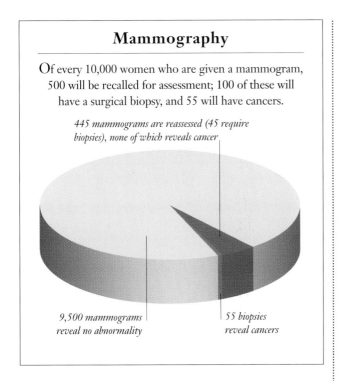

445 mammograms are reassessed (45 require biopsies), none of which reveals cancer

9,500 mammograms reveal no abnormality

55 biopsies reveal cancers

● **Exposure to X-rays might be harmful** Modern screening equipment delivers an extremely low dose of radiation, and, as a result, the chance that mammography could cause a tumor to develop is negligible.

● **Why suffer the concern and discomfort?** On the whole, the negative aspects of having regular mammogram examinations are very clearly outweighed by the real possibility that they could save your life. If you are one of the small minority of women whose mammogram does detect breast cancer, you will have a much better chance of successful treatment and recovery than if the disease remains undiscovered and continues to worsen.

In those women who are screened, three of every ten who would otherwise have died of breast cancer will survive the disease.

KEY POINTS

- The recommendations for regular mammography vary.
- Screening women under the age of 40 or 50 has not been shown to be cost-effective.
- Regular screening allows many breast cancers to be detected at an early stage, when the chances of successful treatment are greatly improved.

Seeing the doctor

Whenever you experience symptoms relating to your breasts, the first person to consult is your gynecologist or primary care physician. His or her priority is to decide whether you might have some serious disease within the breast and, if not, whether the problem can be solved without referring you to another doctor or specialist.

VISITING YOUR DOCTOR
If you have any worries or symptoms relating to your breasts, you should consult your doctor right away.

If you have a definite lump or your doctor wishes to obtain further advice, you may be sent to a breast clinic or breast surgeon. Alternatively, your gynecologist or primary care physician may decide that your breasts should be checked again, perhaps at a different point in your menstrual cycle, and ask you to come back for a follow-up examination. Your doctor might also order a mammogram or ultrasound to further evaluate the problem even in advance of any possible referral.

VISITING A SPECIALIST

The doctor will ask you to describe your symptoms in detail and how long you have had them. If your problem is pain or a lump, he or she will also want to know if it varies in relation to your menstrual cycle. You will then be given a full examination. If you are being checked by a male doctor, he may ask whether you want a female nurse to be present during the examination.

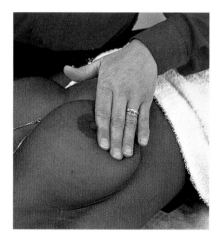

A PHYSICAL EXAMINATION
The doctor will check your breasts for lumps with his or her fingertips.

HAVING A PHYSICAL EXAMINATION

The doctor looks at your breasts with your arms by your side, above your head, and pressing on your hips. Often, by looking carefully at the outline of the breasts in various positions, the doctor can see changes in the outline that will help identify the site and cause of a complaint. The doctor also examines your breasts while you are lying flat with your arms folded under your head.

If the doctor finds a lump during this examination, he or she will concentrate on the area of the lump, examining it with the fingertips and measuring it. After checking the breasts, the doctor usually examines the lymph glands in the armpit and those in the lower part of the neck.

If further investigation is needed, the specialist who sees you will tell you exactly what tests are needed and explain why they are necessary.

MAMMOGRAMS

If you are over 40 and have not had a breast X-ray within the past year, the doctor will probably send you to have one done. This X-ray is known as a mammogram. For more on what happens when you have a mammogram, see pages 15–18. Some doctors may arrange for patients to have mammograms taken before being seen so that the X-rays are on hand when the patients are examined. Otherwise, the film will be ready for the doctor to evaluate soon after the visit.

ULTRASOUND SCANNING

X-rays do not pass easily through the breasts of women who are younger than 35 because their breasts are too dense. This often makes it difficult to obtain images of sufficient quality. Ultrasound, which is familiar to many women because it is used to look at babies during pregnancy, can also be used on the breast to tell whether a lump is solid or filled with fluid (cystic).

Ultrasound is not useful as a screening test; it is of real value only when mammography shows an abnormality or there is unquestionably a lump in the breast. When a lump is solid, ultrasound is an accurate means of judging whether it is benign and straightforward or whether it may be more serious.

NEEDLE TESTS

Inserting a needle into a lump, known as fine needle aspiration (see p.22), can show whether it is a fluid-filled cyst or solid. Since the breast is very sensitive, this test can be uncomfortable, but it does not take long to do.

If the lump is solid, it may be possible to suck out a few cells for microscopic examination to find out whether the lump is benign or cancerous. The needle that is used for these tests is small, the same size as the ones used to take blood.

An alternative, if the doctor is fairly sure that the lump is solid, is to remove a small portion of the lump with a slightly larger needle called a core biopsy needle. Before this test is carried out, the skin and the surrounding tissue are numbed with anesthetic. Provided

What Happens in Fine Needle Aspiration

Fine needle aspiration is a procedure used to withdraw sample cells from a breast lump. A small syringe needle is inserted directly into the lump. If fluid is withdrawn, then the lump is a cyst. If the lump is solid, a sample of cells is removed for microscopic examination.

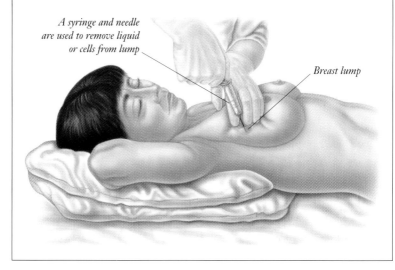

A syringe and needle are used to remove liquid or cells from lump

Breast lump

that the anesthetic has been injected in the right place, it is not a painful test.

When the anesthetic wears off, however, the area where the breast was sampled can be tender. Patients are usually advised to take acetaminophen, ibuprofen, or another analgesic that is used for headaches.

If the doctor finds that there is no serious abnormality in your breast, he or she will reassure you and tell you that you do not have to return for another visit. If the results of a mammography or needle biopsy are not available right away, a follow-up appointment may be needed to discuss them.

Your gynecologist's or primary care physician's office may have a specialist breast-care nurse on the staff. He or she will check to make sure that you understand what the doctor has told you and may help in arranging follow-up appointments and further tests.

FOLLOW-UP

A follow-up appointment will be scheduled if you need to go back to the office to get the results of tests. If they indicate that there is no problem in the breast, you probably will not need to see the doctor again until your next regular checkup. If, however, the tests suggest that the lump might be serious, the doctor will explain what this means.

SEEING A BREAST-CARE NURSE
A specially trained breast-care nurse will explain tests and treatments to you, answer your questions, and discuss concerns that you may have.

Sometimes the results of the tests do not exactly pinpoint what is wrong. In that case you may need to have further investigations.

If you have had a simple needle biopsy that has not shown the cause of the lump, at your second visit you may have a core biopsy, which is described on pages 21–22. Alternatively, a doctor may suggest that the lump be removed. This is called an excisional biopsy, and it can be performed under local anesthesia while you are awake, but it is more commonly done under general anesthesia. Before any operation is performed, you will be asked to sign a consent form agreeing to the removal of the lump. It is important to make sure that the surgeon will remove only that lump and will not

Points of Biopsy Incisions

When a biopsy is carried out, the incision is usually made along natural tension lines in the skin to help keep scarring to a minimum.

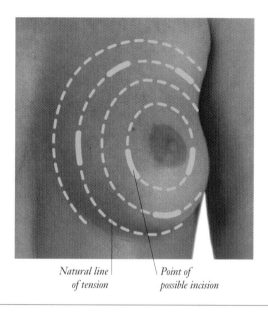

Natural line | Point of
of tension | possible incision

take more tissue without first explaining the procedure and getting your consent.

WHAT DO THE TESTS MEAN?

Needle tests are very accurate, and if the results indicate cancer, they are very rarely wrong. Occasionally, a mammogram or an ultrasound scan is reported as showing a cancer, but, when the site is tested with a needle or removed and analyzed, it turns out to be noncancerous.

This might happen in one out of 20 cases. That is why the doctor will often tell a woman that a lump might be cancer and that it is impossible to be 100 percent certain until the suspect tissue has been removed and analyzed.

The combination of performing a careful examination, doing X-rays and/or scans, and removing cells with a needle for testing is very accurate. If all three of these tests are done, it is very rare to miss a cancer. If all the tests show that a lump is not serious, then it does not necessarily need to be removed.

KEY POINTS

- After examining you, the primary care physician will probably order a mammogram or ultrasound scan or obtain further advice from a specialist.
- The breast specialist will examine you and may perform fine needle aspiration of a breast lump.
- The combination of examination, X-rays or scans, and fine needle aspiration is very accurate in identifying the cause of a breast lump.
- Not all breast lumps need to be removed.

Normal variation in breast development

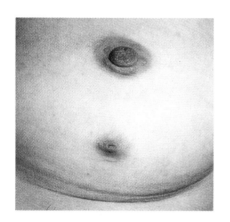

As we saw in the section on developing and changing breasts (pp. 7–8), the ridge of tissue called the milk line normally disappears before birth. Sometimes, however, a part of the ridge that should have disappeared remains and forms an extra nipple or, occasionally, an extra breast.

EXTRA NIPPLE
Some people are born with an extra nipple, which commonly looks like a mole. These can be removed if they cause distress.

Extra nipples are common and between one and four in every 100 people have one. These are usually situated below the normal nipple along the milk line, while extra breasts, if present, are most commonly located in the armpits. These extra nipples or breasts can be affected by the same diseases that affect ordinary breasts. An extra breast that is causing problems, whether physical or psychological, can be surgically removed if necessary.

BREAST SIZE

In theory, breast size does not matter at all; it has no bearing on a woman's sexuality or on her ability to breast-feed. In reality, however, concern about breast size is a source of very real distress to many women. It does not necessarily help them to know that breasts naturally come in many different shapes and sizes or that their own breasts are well within this normal range. It is not at all unusual to have one breast noticeably larger than the other, with a bigger left breast being more common. The difference may not be obvious to anyone else, but, if the discrepancy is very marked, it can be corrected by surgery. Either the smaller breast can be made larger or vice versa.

Having very large breasts can cause women a number of problems. Apart from the possible embarrassment, which can be especially difficult for young women, large breasts may be painful. Their weight puts a strain on the shoulder straps of a bra, which can cut into the skin, and large breasts can cause backaches. They can get in the way of normal physical activity and can be a real handicap when it comes to sports. Any woman troubled by such difficulties should talk them over with her doctor. It may be worth considering surgery to reduce the size of the breasts to improve the woman's quality of life.

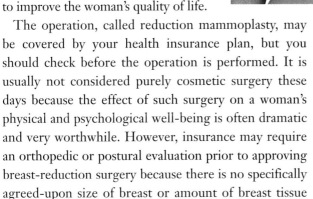

The operation, called reduction mammoplasty, may be covered by your health insurance plan, but you should check before the operation is performed. It is usually not considered purely cosmetic surgery these days because the effect of such surgery on a woman's physical and psychological well-being is often dramatic and very worthwhile. However, insurance may require an orthopedic or postural evaluation prior to approving breast-reduction surgery because there is no specifically agreed-upon size of breast or amount of breast tissue that would automatically require corrective surgery.

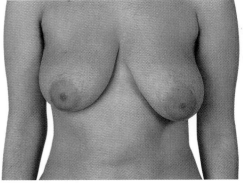

ASYMMETRICAL BREASTS
It is very common for one breast to be larger than the other. The difference is usually not particularly noticeable. If it is, and it causes problems, corrective surgery may be performed.

Breast Reduction Surgery

An operation to reduce the size of the breasts is done under general anesthesia and often takes up to four hours of surgery. It is a fairly major operation and generally involves some degree of discomfort for several days afterward.

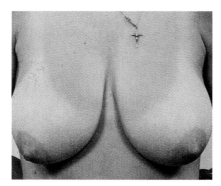

BEFORE SURGERY

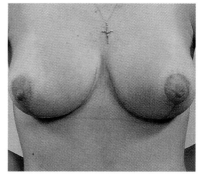

AFTER SURGERY

Having small breasts does not cause the same kind of problems as large ones, although individual women may be very concerned about it. However, since it is extremely rare for insurance companies to consider breast enlargement surgery to be a medical necessity, anyone who wants her breasts enlarged is likely to have to pay for it herself. The possible exception to this rule is reconstruction of a breast after surgery for a lump.

The operation to enlarge the breasts involves inserting implants behind the breast tissue. The most commonly used implants are made of silicone. There was some question about the safety of these silicone implants in the US, but further research has suggested that silicone implants do not do any harm and that there is no reason for women who have them to be concerned.

Alternatives to silicone include saltwater and soybean oil. Neither of these produces as good a result as silicone. Even though the operation to enlarge breasts is not likely to be covered under most health insurance policies, it is still worth asking your doctor for advice if you are considering it because he or she may be able to recommend a good surgeon. It is still possible to breast-feed after you have had breast implants.

The most common complication after insertion of implants is the formation of capsules around the implants. The capsules contract and make the implant harden, which which can cause pain, change of shape, and embarrassment. Rupture of the implants is a major concern among patients. About 10 percent of the earlier varieties with thinner envelopes are liable to rupture after 10 years. However, ruptured implants cause very few problems, because almost all the silicone remains within the fibrous capsule formed by the body. Newer implants are less likely to rupture.

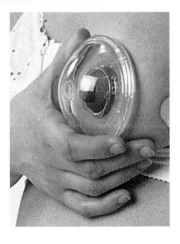

BREAST SHELL
Using a breast shell encourages inverted nipples to protrude, making breast-feeding much easier.

INVERTED NIPPLES

Some women have naturally inverted or "pulled-in" nipples, which causes no significant health problems. However, some of them feel this is an embarrassing "abnormality," and it can cause problems with breast-feeding. Breast "shells" have been reported to be successful in resolving nipple retraction in some women. It is also possible to correct the problem with cosmetic surgery, although the surgery is unlikely to be covered by insurance. During pregnancy, wearing breast shells may encourage the nipples to protrude normally for breast-feeding (see p.46).

29

NIPPLE PIERCING

Cosmetic piercing of the nipples is now fairly common. The ring can damage the ducts underneath the nipple, which can result in recurrent infections or leakage of material from the duct through the skin. If this happens, the ring should be removed and the area allowed to heal.

MALE BREASTS

All men have some breast tissue under the skin. This tissue, like women's, responds to hormonal changes in the body, although much less dramatically. In some cases, particular drugs and occasionally certain illnesses may cause breast swelling. In most people, the situation clears up without the need for anything beyond a medical checkup.

Sometimes, a boy or a grown man starts to develop a breast shape that is like that of a woman. A certain amount of breast development is not uncommon in

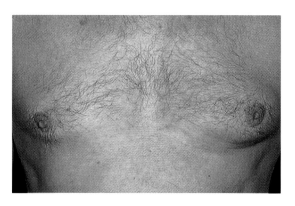

BREASTS IN ELDERLY MEN
Hormonal changes in older men may cause their breasts to grow. Most breast swellings in elderly men are harmless, but a doctor should be consulted.

boys between 10 and 16 years old; it affects between one- and two-thirds of all boys during puberty. This is nothing to worry about, and it will almost certainly disappear naturally in time. However, if it is noticeable enough to be embarrassing or if the swelling has not begun to subside after two years, it is worth seeing your doctor. Breast growth can sometimes occur in middle and later life, and a man between the ages of 50 and 80 who notices breast swelling should tell his doctor. Normally, no treatment is needed, but a mammogram may be necessary to rule out the possibility of a malignant growth. One percent of breast cancers occur in men.

KEY POINTS

- Extra nipples and extra breasts are common.
- Large breasts can cause considerable problems, and surgery to make them smaller is available.
- Small breasts can be made larger using breast implants.
- Enlargement of male breasts, which can be embarrassing, is common in boys between the ages of 10 and 16 but usually disappears within a year or two.

Breast pain

Breast pain is a common problem and can vary with the menstrual cycle. Fortunately, breast pain is amenable to both self-help and pharmacologic therapy.

More often than not, breast pain is not very bad, and many women simply accept it as a normal feature of the changes that are brought on by their menstrual cycle.

Breast pain is rarely a sign of a serious problem. In fact, breast cancer is usually painless. At one time, it was thought that women who were worriers or were depressed were more likely to complain of breast pain. Studies have now shown, however, that there is no connection between mood and breast pain.

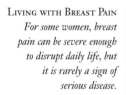

LIVING WITH BREAST PAIN
For some women, breast pain can be severe enough to disrupt daily life, but it is rarely a sign of serious disease.

TYPES OF BREAST PAIN

Breast pain can be divided into two types:
● **Cyclical** This kind of pain is worse immediately before a menstrual period.
● **Noncyclical** In this case, there is no connection between the pain and the time of the month.

If you are uncertain about whether your breast pain follows a regular pattern, it is worth keeping a diary for two or three months. You can ask your doctor for a chart to record your breast pain, or you can simply make your own. You need to note each day how bad the pain is (on a scale from 1 to 5) and mark the days when you have your menstrual period. You could also record other details, such as dietary changes and stressful events. After a while, the diary should help you determine whether your breast pain is cyclical and if there might be other contributing factors for you.

CYCLICAL BREAST PAIN

Symptoms that come and go according to the time of the month are a familiar feature of many women's lives. You may become more aware of your breasts, perhaps because they feel full, heavy, and uncomfortable, or they may become lumpy and tender, usually about 3–7 days before your menstrual period starts. The problem is more common in women in their 30s, but it can also happen in older women if they are using hormone replacement therapy. Although breast pain or tenderness usually disappears after menopause, being pregnant or using oral contraceptives does not generally make a difference, and the discomfort or pain can continue for many years.

You may discover that the pain varies from month to month. Most women describe it as a heaviness or an ache, similar to a toothache, with tenderness experienced when the breast is touched. Certain movements can increase the pain. This is particularly important if a woman's daily activities involve using her arms or lifting a lot. Unless they have experienced it themselves, many people do not realize how severe breast pain can be or how seriously it can affect a woman's life.

KEEPING A DIARY
Writing down incidents of breast pain, making a note of the dates, will help you determine if your breast pain is cyclical or not.

WHAT CAUSES CYCLICAL BREAST PAIN?

Despite the fact that cyclical breast pain occurs each month before a menstrual period, research has failed to show any differences in hormone levels between women who experience bad breast pain and those who do not. Women with breast pain have some abnormality in the level of certain fatty acids in the blood. Lifestyle factors such as smoking, caffeine intake, and diet may play a role, but their contribution is not clear.

CAN IT BE TREATED?

Your doctor will probably want to do a thorough examination to make sure there is nothing seriously wrong. Most women with mild cyclical breast pain do not need specific treatment, but it is worth seeing a trained bra fitter to make sure you are wearing the right size and type of brassiere. A firm, supportive bra of the kind recommended for sports wear can often relieve the pain.

Your doctor can also reassure you that cyclical breast pain has no connection with breast cancer, a fear that is often at the back of many women's minds. Mild breast tenderness that starts just before the menstrual period is due and disappears after it finishes is rarely, if ever, a symptom of any underlying disease.

WEARING A SPORTS BRA
This type of bra will often help alleviate breast pain by providing good support for the breasts.

WILL EVENING PRIMROSE OIL HELP?

If you are one of a modest number of women whose breast pain is so severe that it disrupts your life and interferes with daily activities, your doctor may suggest one of a variety of treatments, one of which is evening primrose oil. The oil is prescribed in a dose of about three grams a day for a trial of three or four months. Over half of those who take it report benefit. If it works, you can consider stopping the treatment after another three months. There is a good chance that the pain will not recur. However, if it does, it may be much less severe. Side effects from evening primrose are few and minor (see the chart on p.39).

WHAT DRUG TREATMENTS ARE AVAILABLE?

A variety of drugs are available that work by interfering with hormones that act on the breast. They include danazol, bromocriptine, and tamoxifen, all of which have side effects. Therefore, it is important to weigh the pros and cons with your doctor before taking them. The side effects, which are summarized in the chart on page 39, disappear when the drug is stopped.

● **Danazol** This often works when evening primrose oil has failed and when the pain is severe. Danazol works by blocking the release of two hormones from the pituitary, which in turn reduces the amount of hormones produced by the ovaries. Levels of circulating estrogen, one of the major hormones thought to cause breast pain, are thereby decreased. However, you cannot take this drug with oral contraceptives, and you must use a mechanical alternative, such as condoms, a coil, or a cap, for contraception.

● **Bromocriptine mesylate** This drug is now rarely used in the treatment of breast pain because of its side effects. It works by reducing the amount of one of the hormones that acts on the breast, prolactin, which plays a role in production of milk. There is now a newer drug

Checking the Fit of Your Bra

Wearing a bra is good for your breasts. When you choose a bra, make sure that it fits correctly and supports your breasts.

- Make sure your bra fits flat around your body and is not too tight. Too tight a fit will be uncomfortable and could cause breathing difficulty. The bra should lie close between your breasts and not stand away from your body.
- See that the breasts are fully contained within each cup; gaping at the side means that the cup is too small. If the cup wrinkles all over, it is too large.
- If the breasts bulge along the top of the cups, the cups are too small.
- Bulges at the armpits indicate that the bra size is too small.
- Check that flesh is not bulging over the top of the cups, under your arms, across the back, or beneath the band.
- If the bra is underwired, the underwiring should lie flat against your body, following the contours of your body, and it should not dig into your breast. A soft-cup bra will fit differently from an underwired bra; the wire contains your breast, whereas the breast can spread in a soft-cup bra.
- If your breasts are heavy, the bra's straps should be wide and strong enough to support them. Make sure that the rest of the bra helps support the breasts.
- The cup spacing should be correct. Make sure your breasts lie naturally, not pushed to one side or the other.
- Always test the fit of your bra both standing and sitting. The breasts tend to "plump up" when you are seated; this is especially noticeable in a strapless bra.

Choosing a Bra

When you choose a bra, make sure that it has adjustable straps and fittings and that it gives you the correct amount of support. Ask for expert advice from a fitting specialist, if necessary.

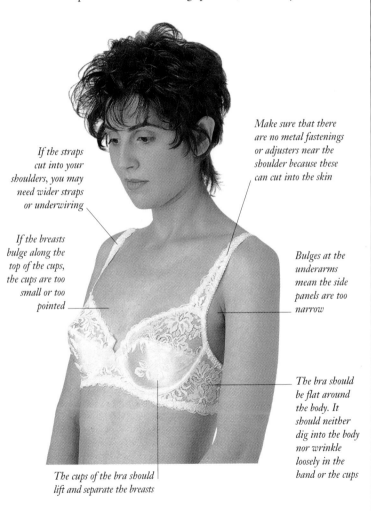

Make sure that there are no metal fastenings or adjusters near the shoulder because these can cut into the skin

If the straps cut into your shoulders, you may need wider straps or underwiring

If the breasts bulge along the top of the cups, the cups are too small or too pointed

Bulges at the underarms mean the side panels are too narrow

The bra should be flat around the body. It should neither dig into the body nor wrinkle loosely in the band or the cups

The cups of the bra should lift and separate the breasts

called cabergoline that reduces the amount of prolactin in the body. This is taken once a week and as yet has not been approved for use in breast pain, but trials are in progress. As with danazol, bromocriptine cannot be used at the same time as oral contraceptives.

● **Tamoxifen** This drug may be used occasionally to treat severe breast pain but only in exceptional circumstances. Tamoxifen interferes with the female hormone estrogen by preventing estrogen from reaching its target cells. It therefore has the same effect as danazol in reducing breast pain.

WHAT OTHER TREATMENTS MIGHT HELP?

Antibiotics, water pills (diuretics), and vitamin B_6 have been used in the past to treat breast pain, but they are now known to be ineffective. Although no particular oral contraceptive has been linked with breast pain, some women find that it helps to change to a brand with a lower level of progesterone. Others find that the pain lessens if they stop taking oral contraceptives altogether and begin to use an alternative means of contraception. Starting hormone replacement therapy (HRT) can sometimes bring on breast pain and lumpiness. This usually improves over time, but it can remain a problem for some women. In these women, evening primrose oil is generally effective in controlling the pain and lumpiness.

HOW CAN YOU HELP YOURSELF?

Keep a diary to record when your pain comes and goes and note any factors that seem to influence it. Try the various strategies listed opposite one at a time and see whether or not each one helps. If you try them

Possible Side Effects of Treatments

All the side effects of breast pain treatment are reversible – that is, they disappear when the treatment is stopped – but you will not necessarily get any or all of them.

TREATMENT	POSSIBLE SIDE EFFECTS
Evening primrose oil	Occasional: stomach upset, greasy skin and hair
Danazol	Oily skin, acne occasionally, and occasional deepening of the voice
Bromocriptine	Nausea, light-headedness
Tamoxifen	Hot flashes

all at once, you will not know which ones led to any improvement in your pain.

● Get your bra size checked by a trained fitter; buy a couple of supportive, sports-style bras; and, when your breasts are painful, wear a bra day and night.

● Start doing regular aerobic exercise.

● If you are a smoker, stop.

● Experiment with your diet. Some women find that avoiding fried and fatty foods and drinks containing caffeine and cutting down on salt can all be helpful in relieving breast pain.

NONCYCLICAL BREAST PAIN

Women who experience this type of breast pain tend to be older than those whose pain is cyclical, with an average age of 43. The pain of noncyclical mastalgia can

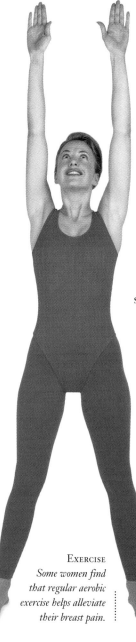

arise from the breast itself, from the muscles and ribs under the breast, or from areas outside the breast.

You may feel the pain as one or more tender spots over your ribs, next to the breastbone, or over the ribs just outside your breast. This type of pain actually comes from the muscles or the ribs. It may be constant, but more often, it comes and goes without any regular pattern. Women usually describe the pain as burning or pulling, but it can sometimes be stabbing in nature.

CAN TREATMENT HELP?

Before the doctor can offer you any treatment, he or she needs to identify precisely where your pain is coming from. If the source can be pinpointed to a specific area on the chest wall, you may be given simple analgesics, an anti-inflammatory cream or gel to rub in, or an injection of a local anesthetic and a steroid.

Noncyclical pain coming from the breast itself is often eased by a simple analgesic, such as ibuprofen. Wearing a well-fitting supportive bra day and night can also help. If these simple measures do not work, your doctor may think it worthwhile to try evening primrose oil (see pp.34–35). Although these options do not work as well as for women with cyclical breast pain and only about half as many women respond to treatment, they have very few side effects.

The drugs used for cyclical breast pain, such as danazol, can also be tried in extreme cases. Unfortunately, they do not work as often for noncyclical pain, and they have more side effects than evening primrose oil (see p.39).

EXERCISE
Some women find that regular aerobic exercise helps alleviate their breast pain.

KEY POINTS

- Breast pain is very common.
- It is not often a symptom in women with breast cancer.
- Wearing a firm supportive bra can help relieve the pain.
- Pain that comes and goes in relation to the menstrual cycle usually responds to treatment.
- Hormone replacement therapy can cause breast pain in older women.
- Pain that is not related to the menstrual cycle is best treated by simple analgesics.

Breast infection

Breast infections most often affect women between the ages of 18 and 50. However, they are much less common than they used to be. Although breast infections can occur at any time, many happen while a woman is breast-feeding her baby.

BREAST-FEEDING INFECTIONS
Nipple infections in lactating mothers are common during the early weeks of breast-feeding. The breast becomes hot, red, and painful.

BREAST-FEEDING

Infection is most likely to be a problem during the first six weeks of breast-feeding, although some women develop it while they are weaning their babies. Although it can be treated effectively, it is far better to prevent it. If you have problems getting your baby to breast-feed happily and comfortably, seek the advice of your midwife, breast-feeding counselor, or obstetrician.

The first symptoms of a breast infection are pain, swelling, redness, and tenderness, and you may start to feel sick, with a fever, general aches and pains, and a headache, almost as though you had the flu. Before the infection developed, you may have been aware of a cracked nipple or a break in the nearby skin. Infection is more likely when the breasts become engorged with milk that does not drain properly. The milk flow that normally washes away any harmful bacteria is therefore reduced. Many mothers find that their babies feed more easily from one breast than from the other. Often it is the left breast if the mother is right-handed, and vice versa. This can mean that the "less popular" breast is not completely emptied and is thus more prone to engorgement and infection.

If you suspect that you have an infection, you should see your doctor as soon as you can. You will probably be given a prescription for one of the antibiotics that can be taken safely while breast-feeding. It is important that you continue feeding your baby from the infected breast because draining the milk from it completely will reduce the chances of an abscess forming. Your baby will not be harmed by the bacteria in your milk because they are killed by acid in his or her stomach. If you cannot continue feeding for any reason, you should express the milk from the infected breast, either by hand or by using a breast pump.

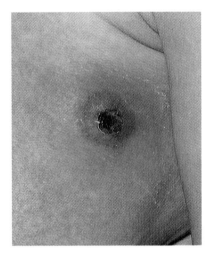

If the infection does not clear up quickly on antibiotics, it is possible that an abscess has formed, and your doctor may decide to send you to a surgeon. Drainage of the abscess can often be done in the office under local anesthesia. In some cases, general anesthesia is needed. A fine needle is used to withdraw the contents of the abscess, which is a localized collection of pus. Sometimes this procedure, called fine needle aspiration (see p.22), needs to be repeated. Until recently, an abscess would have been opened surgically, and this method is still used in some cases. Once the abscess has been drained, you can resume breast-feeding from that breast.

BREAST ABSCESS
An abscess is a collection of pus in the tissue and is caused by an infection. An abscess may cause tenderness and, if it is close to the skin, inflammation.

OTHER BREAST INFECTIONS

Women who are not breast-feeding sometimes develop an infection, usually in an area close to the nipple. Most of them are in their late twenties or early thirties, and about 90 percent of them are smokers. Something in cigarette smoke damages the major ducts beneath the nipple, and the damaged area can then become infected. The condition, known as periductal mastitis, causes pain and redness in the area around the nipple, and sometimes there is an underlying lump.

Normally, antibiotics cure the infection, but if not, an abscess may have developed. When this happens, you will need to have the abscess drained (see p.43).

Unfortunately, because draining the abscess does not remove the damaged duct, the problem may recur. Sometimes, the duct is so severely damaged that a hole develops that allows fluid from the duct to leak through the skin and prevents healing. This condition is known as a mammary duct fistula. If you develop this problem or suffer repeated bouts of infection, you may need a minor operation to remove the damaged ducts.

A woman may, less commonly, develop an infection in a part of the breast away from the nipple. This type of infection usually responds well to antibiotic treatment.

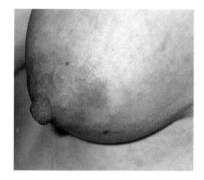

PERIDUCTAL MASTITIS
Nonlactational mastitis causes pain and redness around the nipple. It is more common in women who smoke than in nonsmokers.

SKIN INFECTIONS

Some women who have large breasts may find that the skin on the underside of their breasts becomes infected. These infections develop because the skin of the breasts is in constant contact with the skin of the chest wall or abdomen, which produces heat and sweating. Consequently, the skin in this area becomes an ideal breeding ground for bacteria and fungi.

Usually, the problem can be treated with an antibiotic or antifungal cream that you rub into the affected area. You will be advised to keep it as clean and dry as possible by washing twice a day and gently drying the skin by dabbing it with a cotton towel or using a hair dryer. You should avoid using talc or body lotion and wear either cotton bras or a cotton undershirt between the bra and the skin. If the cream and hygiene measures do not work, it may indicate that you have a more serious infection requiring treatment with oral antibiotics. If you are overweight, you can reduce the chances of recurrent infection by losing weight. However, if your weight is normal and you simply have very large breasts, it may be worth considering whether you could benefit from surgery to make them smaller (see pp.27–28).

KEY POINTS

- Breast infection during breast-feeding is now uncommon but can be a problem, particularly during the first six weeks.
- If you suspect that you have an infection, visit your doctor as soon as possible for antibiotics. You can continue to breast-feed even if you are taking antibiotics.
- Infection around the nipple in nonlactating women is associated with smoking.

Nipple problems

Problems with nipples are relatively common, but fortunately, most of them are not serious.

PREPARING FOR FEEDING
Pregnant women who have inverted nipples and wish to breast-feed may benefit from wearing breast shells inside their bra.

NIPPLE SHAPE

Some women's nipples are naturally retracted, but this is not usually a problem unless you want to breast-feed. Wearing breast shells inside your bra while you are pregnant will encourage your nipples to protrude and thereby make feeding your baby easier.

If your nipples change shape and retract or become pulled to one side as you get older, you should let your doctor know. This is often just a normal feature of aging because the major ducts under the nipples get shorter and wider. As they become shorter, they pull the middle part of the nipple in, producing a slit effect across the nipple. Sometimes the ducts fill up with a cheesy substance that may leak out through the nipples (see p.48). Your doctor will probably want you to be examined and have a mammogram to make sure everything is normal and there is no lump behind the nipple. Occasionally, a pulled-in nipple may be a sign of inflammation in the ducts underneath the nipple. For women whose nipples change shape or become indrawn, a mammogram (and possibly an ultrasound) is usually necessary to exclude the possibility of cancer. Once any serious underlying disease has been ruled out, they can rest assured that the change in their nipple shape is nothing they need to worry about.

NIPPLE DISCHARGE

Discharge usually comes through the nipple from the ducts underneath. However, it may sometimes come from the surface of the nipple itself. Two-thirds of women who are not pregnant can be made to produce fluid from the nipple simply by cleaning it and massaging the breast. A common form of discharge is a milky fluid that can continue to leak from the breasts for months or even years after a woman has finished feeding her baby. More rarely, a woman may produce milk from her nipples even though she is not and has never been pregnant.

All women, even if they have never been pregnant, have fluid inside their breasts. This fluid does not normally find its way to the outside because the ducts are blocked with plugs of a substance called keratin. Vigorous exercise or sexual activity may dislodge these plugs and release fluid in a discharge that comes and goes. The fluid may come from one or both breasts and usually appears only in small amounts. It may range in color from white to pale yellow to green to blue-black. In all cases, it is perfectly normal.

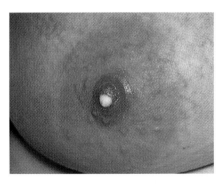

MILKY DISCHARGE
The breasts can sometimes secrete milk in a woman who is not breast-feeding.

Discharge that is caused by duct disease tends to be more troublesome, appears in larger quantities, and is present all the time. Yellowish or blood-stained discharge is most likely to be caused by a benign growth, known

47

as a papilloma, in one of the ducts beneath the nipple. Discharges that are blood-stained, persistent, or troublesome are easily treated by removing the abnormal duct. This is a simple operation and is performed through a small incision around the nipple.

A thicker, cheesy discharge can occur in older women whose ducts widen with age. The ducts become filled with cheesy material that can leak out onto the surface of the nipple.

It is also possible to suffer from a discharge from the skin surrounding the nipple rather than from the nipple itself. Some women have trouble with eczema on the areola, the skin around the nipple. Although the cause is not clear, treatment with a topical steroid cream is usually effective.

Another possible cause of discharge is a disease of the skin of the nipple known as Paget's disease of the nipple. This causes an ulcer on the surface of the nipple. It is usually a sign of cancer or precancer present in the breast.

Women who have a discharge from the surface of the nipple or the surrounding skin need a careful breast examination and mammography. If necessary, samples of skin and tissue from the breast

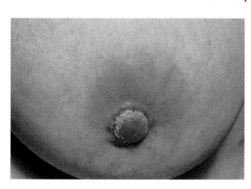

PAGET'S DISEASE
This rare form of nipple crusting involves the milk ducts of the nipple.

may be taken for microscopic examination. If tests show Paget's disease of the nipple, an operation is usually required. The surgery may entail removal of only the nipple and the tissue underneath it and may be followed by radiation therapy, or a mastectomy may be required (see pp.66–69).

KEY POINTS

- Problems with the nipples are common.
- Pulling in of the nipple can be the result of infection, aging, or cancer.
- Most discharges from the nipple are not serious.

Breast lumps

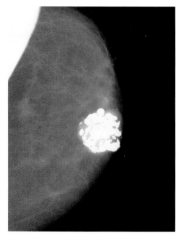

A BENIGN TUMOR
This mammogram shows a fibroadenoma, a noncancerous tumor. Fibroadenomas commonly arise in the breasts of women under the age of 20.

*M*ost breast lumps are not cancerous. In fact, most women have lumpy breasts, and many of the lumps they find are just lumpy areas of normal breast tissue that become more prominent. This type of lump is often easier to feel in the few days just before your menstrual period is due.

At one time, women with lumpy breasts were said to have fibrocystic disease. Having lumpy breasts does not make a woman more likely to develop breast cancer. However, if you notice a new, distinct, and separate lump in your breast, you should discuss it promptly with your doctor.

FIBROADENOMAS

Strictly speaking, fibroadenomas are not a disease at all. They are overgrowths of the "leaves," or breast lobules, described on pages 8–10. They account for six out of 10 lumps found in women under the age of 20 and are relatively uncommon later in life. Ultrasound and fine needle aspiration (see pp.21–23) are usually used to confirm the diagnosis. Once your doctor has determined that the lump is a fibroadenoma, you may not need treatment. At least one in three such lumps shrink or disappear on their own within two years.

However, if you are worried about the lump or if it is growing, you can choose to have it removed.

CYSTS

Cysts are swollen lobules that can form as breast tissue ages. They usually affect women in their 30s, 40s, and 50s. The development of cysts is especially common during the years just before menopause. Although researchers do not know what causes cysts, they do know it is not just a blockage of a duct.

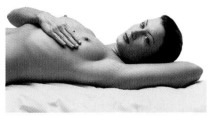

Most cysts are smooth, mobile lumps. Some are large enough to be easily visible, and they can be painful. It is usually very easy for doctors to identify a cyst with ultrasound and, in some cases, with mammography. The final and definitive investigation is also the treatment for a cyst. The doctor inserts a fine needle into the lump without anesthesia and extracts the fluid from inside the cyst. Usually, the lump disappears completely. The fluid may be yellow, green, or blue-black. If the fluid is blood-stained, it is sent for tests because, rarely, a cancer may form in the wall of a cyst. Although such cancers are rare, cysts that produce blood-stained fluid are usually removed.

Of every six women who develop a cyst, three will never have another one. Two of the six will have three to five cysts during their lifetime, and the remaining woman will have more than five. It is not necessary to have all cysts drained, provided that the doctor is confident that a cyst is present rather than a solid lump. Women who have had one or more cysts are not at significantly increased risk of developing breast cancer.

BREAST LUMPS
If you notice a lump in your breast, it is likely to be one of the two common benign types: a fibroadenoma or a cyst. These lumps, which are harmless, are part of the normal changing growth pattern of breasts.

KEY POINTS

- Most lumps are not cancerous.
- The most common type of lump in a young woman is a fibroadenoma.
- Fibroadenomas may not need to be removed.
- Cysts are more common in women in their 30s, 40s, and 50s. They are treated by inserting a fine needle and removing the fluid.
- Benign lumps are not associated with a significantly increased risk of breast cancer.

Breast cancer

More women get breast cancer than any other type of cancer: about one in 12 will have the disease at some point in her life. A woman's risk of developing breast cancer doubles every 10 years, but it is actually very rare in younger women.

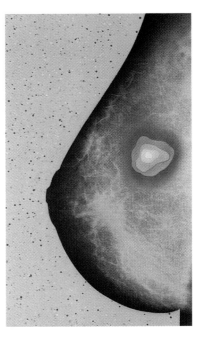

Although breast cancer is the most common cause of death in women between the ages of 35 and 50, many women, including those under the age of 50, are correctly diagnosed with and successfully treated for the disease. It is also worth remembering that nine out of 10 breast lumps are found to be benign, or noncancerous, and that breast cancer is relatively rare in younger women. The earlier that malignant, or cancerous, lumps are detected and treated, the better the woman's chances of survival.

EARLY DETECTION
This color-enhanced mammogram reveals the presence of a breast tumor, seen here as a yellow area. The earlier cancer is detected, the better the chance of long-term survival.

WHY IS CANCER A PROBLEM?

A lot of cells in the human body are growing at any one time, but their growth is very carefully controlled so that the number of cells that are produced matches the number of cells that are dying. A cancer consists of cells that are growing and dividing at a faster rate than cells are dying. The group of cells that form the lump gets bigger and bigger. As the lump increases in size, some of the cells develop the ability to move away from the lump and spread to other parts of the body through the blood-stream or lymphatic channels. This spreading is called metastasis of a cancer. Some of the cells that get into the bloodstream start to form new lumps in different areas of the body. This can cause major problems if the cancer cells grow in important areas, such as the lungs, liver, or brain, or if the cells involve many different bones.

WHAT ARE THE RISK FACTORS?

It is not a simple matter to try to work out your personal level of risk because so many factors play a part in determining who gets breast cancer. In any case, an individual woman has little or no control over most of the risk factors. If you face a higher than average risk, it is important to take advantage of screening programs and visit your doctor promptly if you suspect that you may have a problem.

Even if you know you are more susceptible to breast cancer than other women, any lump you find is still more likely to be benign than malignant.

Experts have worked out some of the factors that increase the risk of developing breast cancer. Remember, though, that even if a woman has all of these factors, she still might not develop breast cancer.

● **Getting older** The chances of developing breast cancer double every 10 years.

● **When your periods begin and end** Starting early or continuing beyond age 55 is linked with increased risk.

● **Postponing pregnancy** Women who do not become pregnant until after the age of 30, or who never have children, are at greater risk than those who are pregnant for the first time at a younger age.

- **Breast-feeding** A woman who has breast-fed one or more children may have a lower risk than a woman who has never done so.

- **Abnormal breast cells** Certain breast conditions may make later cancer more likely. For example, women who have had previous biopsies that show atypical hyperplasia, which is also known as lobular carcinoma in situ (LCIS), will need regular checkups. Other types of noncancerous breast problems do not increase your risk of developing cancer in the future.

- **Overweight** Being seriously overweight, more than 1.5 times the average weight for your height, increases breast cancer risk.

- **Drinking and smoking** Some studies have shown a link between drinking alcohol and breast cancer, and women who drink a lot have a higher risk than those who either drink no alcohol or drink it in moderation. Smoking has not been directly linked to breast cancer risk, but its contribution to other diseases and its negative effects on your general well-being cannot be overemphasized.

- **Oral contraceptives** There is a very slightly increased risk for women while they are taking oral forms of contraception. The risk is short-lived and disappears 10 years after stopping medication.

- **Hormone replacement therapy** For the first 10 years of hormone replacement therapy (HRT), the health benefits outweigh the slightly increased risk of breast cancer. But after that, the risk becomes more important. For a woman of 50, over the next 20 years

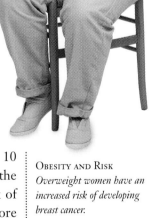

OBESITY AND RISK
Overweight women have an increased risk of developing breast cancer.

she has a one-in-22 chance of developing breast cancer that increases to one in 20 if she uses hormone replacement therapy for 10 years. The risk goes up to one in 17–18 for 15 years of use.

The decision of whether to remain on hormone replacement therapy for more than 10 years is an individual one and is based on the pros and cons for each individual woman. HRT is usually given to a woman with a strong family history of breast cancer only if she is experiencing major problems with menopause.

Relationship of HRT to Breast Cancer Development

The incidence of breast cancer among women over 50 who are using HRT increases with the length of treatment.

TIME ON HRT	EXTRA CANCERS IN HRT USERS
None	–
5 years	2 per 1,000
10 years	6 per 1,000
15 years	12 per 1,000

● **Family history** One in 10 women who develop breast cancer have inherited some kind of genetic abnormality that makes them more susceptible to the condition. There are various ways of identifying women with this kind of risk, detailed in the box on the opposite page.

If you are seeing your doctor about a breast problem and know that several members of your family have had some form of cancer, you should find out as much as you can about the details of your family history. It would be useful to know what type of cancer they had, at what ages they developed it, and, if relevant, at what ages they died.

Cancer genes can be inherited from either parent, even though neither of them may have actually developed cancer themselves. No one yet knows how many breast cancer genes there are, but five have been identified so far.

Breast Cancer Families

Some women have a greater than average chance of developing breast cancer due to some abnormality in their genetic makeup. The risk may be increased if any of the following apply:

- Several members of a woman's family have or have had breast cancer.
- She has relatives who developed breast cancer while under the age of 50. The earlier in life it happened, the greater the risk that it was caused by an inherited abnormality.
- She has relatives who while young had cancer in both breasts or had certain other types of cancer, particularly cancer of the ovaries, colon, or prostate, which can be caused by the same gene that causes breast cancer.

About one in three cases of inherited breast cancer is thought to be due to an abnormality in a gene known as BRCA-1 and the same proportion to another gene called BRCA-2. The other three genes and a number of undiscovered genes are believed to be responsible for the remaining one-third. Testing for abnormal genes is currently available only in certain laboratories.

Women who come from such affected families may be given the opportunity to find out if they are carrying the abnormal gene and are at increased risk. Women who carry an abnormal gene have a 50–80 percent chance of actually developing breast cancer at some time.

Before opting for the genetic test, women should be aware that, if they are found to have an abnormal gene, it could be difficult for them to obtain life insurance. Consequently, women who do have the genetic test are offered counseling both before and after.

If a woman does carry an abnormal gene, she can take steps to reduce the risk of actually developing breast

Family History and Incidence of Breast Cancer

Breast cancer can affect successive generations of women in a single family, suggesting the presence of a strong hereditary factor. Given her family history, the woman at the bottom of this family tree has decided to undergo genetic tests.

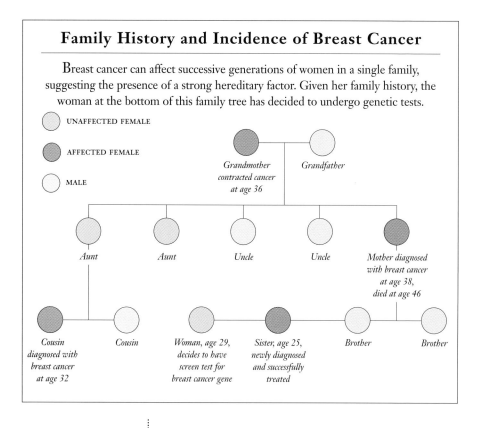

cancer. Usually this involves starting regular intensive screening at an earlier age. Women whose family history suggests that they are at very high risk or those who carry a cancer-related gene can opt for a double mastectomy with or without breast reconstruction. Alternatively, they can participate in one of the ongoing drug studies to try to prevent breast cancer from developing.

As you can see, there is not much anyone can do to eliminate many of the risk factors. However, it is worth trying to get your weight down if you need to and reducing the amount of alcohol in your diet.

How Is a Diagnosis Made?

A woman may notice a lump or change in a breast, or signs of a problem may be picked up by her doctor or on a routine mammogram. It is very important to be aware of how your breasts normally feel and look so that you will notice a change right away. Of course, you must follow up such observations by going to your gynecologist or primary care physician.

Any woman who finds a lump or other abnormality in her breast is bound to be worried, but, the sooner you get it properly checked out, the better.

The chapter Seeing the doctor (see pp.19–25) explains in detail what happens when you go for an examination and what tests may be required when you have a breast problem that needs investigation. The flow chart (see p.11) summarizes the various stages of such an evaluation.

KEY POINTS

- Breast cancer affects one in 12 women in the US.
- A woman's chance of getting breast cancer doubles every 10 years of her life.
- Up to 10 percent of women with breast cancer have a gene that increases the risk of developing the condition.
- Screening is recommended at a younger age for women at high risk.
- Genetic testing is widely available but should not be performed without counseling.
- For the first 10 years of using hormone replacement therapy, its benefits outweigh the slightly increased risk of developing breast cancer.

Extent and kinds of breast cancer

*M*any people do not realize that breast cancer is not just one disease that is always treated in the same way and that has the same predictable outlook for everyone who gets it.

There are several aspects of breast cancer that play a part in determining how well a woman will do and whether her outlook is likely to be better or worse. Factors that must be taken into consideration include the size of the tumor, its potential to spread outside the breast, and what it looks like under the microscope.

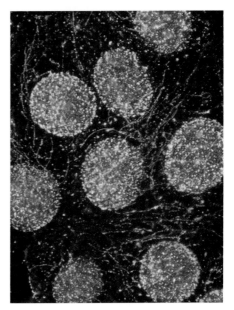

CANCER CELLS
This light micrograph shows cultured human breast cancer cells, magnified 64 times.

ASSESSING THE PROBLEM

Breast cancers develop from the cells that line the breast lobules and the draining ducts. Cancer cells that are confined to the lobule and the ducts are called in situ or noninvasive. They are also sometimes referred to as precancers, since they are not able to spread to other parts of the body. An invasive breast cancer is one in

61

which the cells have moved beyond the ducts and lobules into the surrounding breast tissue.

Noninvasive cancer can turn into invasive cancer if left untreated. Invasive cancers have the ability to spread. They most commonly enter lymph channels in the breast and spread to the lymph glands under the arm, or they can get into the bloodstream to spread elsewhere in the body. The lymph system, a network of lymph channels and lymph glands throughout the body, is primarily involved in fighting infection. Since the lymph glands that drain the breast are under the arms, cancer cells, like bacteria, can travel through these channels to the lymph glands.

Both noninvasive and invasive cancers are further subdivided according to other criteria. In the case of invasive cancers, the most important distinctions are in the different ways they grow and spread and the type of cells involved.

When a cancer is examined under the microscope, it may be possible to determine how aggressive the cancer is likely to be, in other words, how far and how fast it is likely to spread. Once this type of analysis has been done, a tumor may be designated grade I, grade II, or grade III, in order of seriousness.

Rather than being a single disease, breast cancer is in fact a number of separate diseases. At one end of the spectrum is a small cancer consisting of a special type of cell that is easy to control. At the other extreme is a large cancer that has cells of no special type. This type of cancer may be more difficult to treat. The aim is always to determine what type of tumor an individual has in order to tailor the treatment to the specific type of cancer.

Before the doctors decide on the treatment, they need to know whether the cancer has spread and, if so, how far. Normally, if breast cancer is diagnosed, you will be given a thorough clinical examination, blood tests, and a chest X-ray to see if there is evidence of cancer elsewhere in the body and to check your general fitness for surgery.

Occasionally, the doctor may decide to do a bone scan to check all of your bones and a liver scan to look in detail at your liver. The results may provide additional information that allows the doctor to assess the stage of the cancer and the best way to treat it.

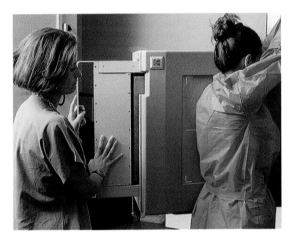

HAVING A CHEST X-RAY
Before starting any treatment for breast cancer, you will have a general examination, including a chest X-ray.

This process, which is known as "staging" the cancer, distinguishes three main groups.

- **Early** This term describes cancer that appears to be confined to the breast and/or the lymph nodes of the armpit on the same side of the body. After the tumor has been surgically removed, radiation therapy is given, and sometimes followed by hormonal therapy or chemotherapy.
- **Locally advanced** Cancer that has not apparently spread beyond the breast and armpit but consists of larger tumors, more extensive involvement of the lymph nodes, or involvement of the skin of the breast. Locally advanced cancers are usually treated with chemotherapy first to shrink the tumor, followed by surgery and radiation therapy.

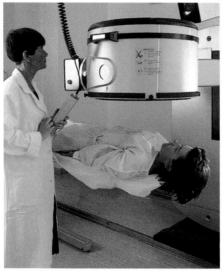

- **Advanced** Chemotherapy and radiation therapy are the primary treatments. However, surgery may be needed to reduce the size of large tumors in the breast to provide comfort and improve appearance.

CANCER SPREAD
Scanning with a gamma camera is a technique used to look for evidence of spread of the cancer to other parts of the body.

KEY POINTS

- There are many different types of breast cancer.
- Cancer cells confined to lobules and breast ducts are called in situ or precancer.
- The most common site for an invasive cancer to spread is the lymph nodes under the arm.

Treating breast cancer

Once a thorough assessment has been made, it is possible to work out the most appropriate treatment. This might include surgery, radiation therapy, hormone therapy, chemotherapy, or a combination, depending on the cancer itself and the patient's wishes.

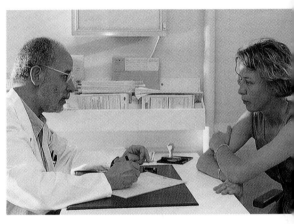

TREATMENT OPTIONS
It is very important to discuss all treatment options with your doctor once breast cancer has been diagnosed.

After the various treatment options have been explained to you, you will be invited to share in the decision-making about what treatments are used. However, some women prefer to leave such decisions to their doctors.

In most cases, treatment is likely to involve surgery alone or surgery and radiation therapy to deal with the cancer in the breast and the glands under the arm. This may be followed by drug treatment aimed at destroying any undetected cancer cells that may have escaped into other parts of the body.

Of all the types of cancer, breast cancer is one of the most treatable, and it is associated with a high cure rate. Despite the fact that more women develop breast cancer every year, the number who actually die from breast cancer is falling, which demonstrates the effectiveness of current treatments.

SURGICAL REMOVAL

When the cancer is relatively small (less than 1½in/ 4cm in size), it is usually possible for the surgeon to remove it along with a small amount of surrounding tissue. This approach is known as breast-conserving surgery, or lumpectomy. However, if the breast is relatively small or if the lump is larger than 1½in (4cm) in size, this breast-conserving operation may not be feasible because so much of the breast has to be removed to get rid of the cancer.

In fact, about one in three breast cancers cannot be removed conservatively and are best treated with mastectomy, an operation to remove the entire breast, usually including the nipple. Fortunately, surgical technique has improved dramatically since the days when a radical mastectomy was the most common procedure. In a radical mastectomy, all the tissue is removed, right down to the chest wall, leaving the woman with a serious deformity of the chest and arm and damaging her ability to use her arm normally. Today, simple mastectomy involves removal of the breast without taking as much under-lying tissue. Some women actually choose to have a mastectomy even though they could have a simple lump removal. In addition, there are certain situations in which a woman with a lump smaller than 1½in (4cm) may be advised to have a mastectomy.

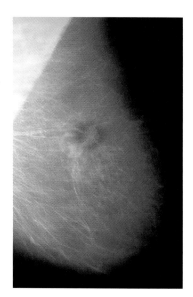

SAVING THE BREAST
This mammogram shows a small, cancerous breast tumor. Small lumps such as this can often be surgically removed, leaving the breast intact.

Different Types of Breast Surgery

The extent of surgery necessary in breast cancer depends on the size, location, outline, and nature of the cancerous tumor. A surgeon will attempt to remove the minimum amount of tissue necessary to remove all of the cancer.

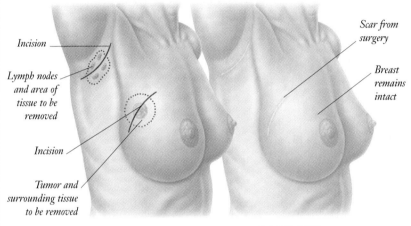

Incision

Lymph nodes and area of tissue to be removed

Incision

Tumor and surrounding tissue to be removed

Scar from surgery

Breast remains intact

BREAST-CONSERVING SURGERY: BEFORE AND AFTER

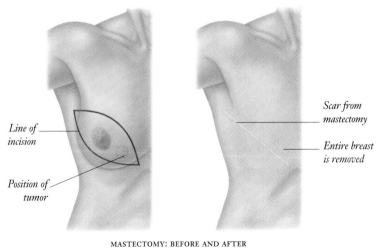

Line of incision

Position of tumor

Scar from mastectomy

Entire breast is removed

MASTECTOMY: BEFORE AND AFTER

The major situations of this kind are:

- When there is more than one lump in the breast. Research shows that even if all these lumps are removed, other cancerous lumps are likely to develop later in other parts of the same breast.
- When the cancer is directly under the nipple and the nipple would have to be removed at the same time. Rather than leave the breast without a nipple, it is sometimes better to remove the breast altogether and have a breast reconstruction (see pp.69–72).
- Sometimes, an operation to remove the lump is not entirely successful. Some cancer or precancer is left behind. Another operation to remove more tissue may solve the problem, or it may be necessary to remove the entire breast.
- Sometimes, the tissue surrounding the lump is abnormal and on its way to becoming cancerous. If it cannot all be removed with a wide excision, a mastectomy may be the safest option.

The surgeon normally removes some of the lymph glands from under the arm. These glands are the most common place to which the cancer may spread. Knowing whether this has happened and, if so, how many of the glands are affected is important both in assessing the severity of the cancer and in deciding on drug treatment. If the surgeon just needs to see whether the cancer has moved into these glands, removing either a single gland that drains the cancer or a few of them is usually sufficient. If tests on one or only a few of the glands that were removed show that they have been affected by cancer, the remaining lymph glands need to be treated with radiation therapy. Most women undergo a course of radiation therapy after breast-conservation surgery even if the glands are not affected (see the section on radiation therapy, pp.72–73).

Sometimes, underarm surgery can cause damage to the nerves in the upper arm, making the armpit feel numb afterward. This is obviously a nuisance but usually does not last long. About one in 20 women who have all their lymph glands removed or who have had them treated with radiation therapy develop lymphedema, or swelling in the arm. Treatment can usually reduce the problem, although it cannot always be eliminated completely. Massage and wearing an elastic stocking can help. You should prop your arm up on several pillows while you are sitting. It is also important to avoid injury or infection in your hand because either can result in worse swelling after the injury has healed or the infection has cleared.

BREAST RECONSTRUCTION

If you have decided with your doctor on a mastectomy, the surgeon will likely discuss with you the possibility of having breast reconstruction surgery done at the same time. The operation is often more successful if done immediately than if delayed for several months. There is no evidence that immediate reconstruction makes a recurrence of cancer any more likely or that, if it does recur, it will be harder to detect.

HOW IS RECONSTRUCTION DONE?

The simplest method is to insert an implant under the skin. This usually needs to be combined with some means of stretching the remaining skin to make up for the amount that was removed during the mastectomy. The procedure may be done in two stages, expanding

Breast Reconstruction Using Implant

After breast surgery, a patient may opt for reconstructive surgery. One type of surgery involves inserting an implant under the skin. This is expanded over several months by injecting saline solution into it.

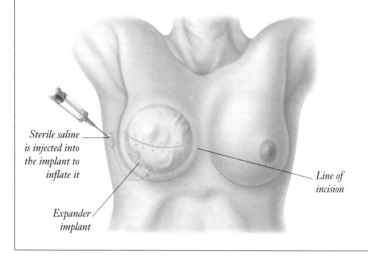

Sterile saline is injected into the implant to inflate it

Line of incision

Expander implant

the skin before inserting the implant, or a combined expander and implant can be used. The expander is gradually inflated with injections of fluid over a period of months to stretch the skin. When the process is complete and the skin has expanded enough, the device can either be removed and replaced with a permanent prosthesis or implant, or some fluid can be removed, leaving the smaller, breast-size implant in position.

Most implants consist of a plastic shell or envelope that is filled with silicone gel or saline solution. Older implants had a very thin shell, and small amounts of silicone occasionally leaked out of them. The newer implants have a much thicker outer shell, so they are much less likely to leak any silicone. The body produces tissue, or a capsule, around an implant. Even if the implant does leak silicone, in all but a few women all of the silicone remains within this capsule. Very occasionally, the silicone can leak into the surrounding tissues, where it can cause irritation and scarring.

Many medical devices placed into the body, including artificial joints and heart valves, contain silicone. Silicone that gets into the bloodstream can occasionally find its way to other parts of the body, but even at this stage it does not seem to cause significant problems. There is, for instance, no evidence now that silicone, when it leaks, causes joint problems or any other disease. Alternative implants are available that contain saltwater or soybean oil. About one woman in 10 experiences problems with implants because the capsule around the implant tightens or hardens and causes the implant to change shape, and this may be painful.

The original implants had a smooth surface, but the newer implants have a rough, irregular (textured) surface. These textured prostheses are associated with a much lower incidence of hardening.

Occasionally an infection may develop, although the chances of this happening are considerably reduced by administering antibiotics to the woman both during and after the operation.

An alternative to using artificial implants alone is to bring skin and muscle from another part of the body to replace the lost breast. These tissues may be taken from the back or the abdomen. The "back flap" method uses a muscle called the latissimus dorsi. With this procedure, an implant is usually needed in addition to the muscle to create the appropriate-size breast.

When the muscle from the abdomen is used, it is sometimes possible to transfer fat as well, making an implant unnecessary.

The main disadvantage of using transplanted tissue is that it does not always survive. About one in every 100 back-flap and one in every 20 abdominal-flap operations fail for this reason.

Whether the surgeon uses muscle or an implant to reconstruct the breast, it is possible to construct a nipple at a later time. This is done either by transplanting some darker-colored skin from the upper inner thigh or by tattooing the skin to create an areola. A simpler solution is to opt for one of the very natural-looking stick-on nipples now available.

RADIATION THERAPY

There is good evidence to show that all women who have had breast-conserving surgery benefit from radiation therapy treatment afterward. However, only about one-quarter of mastectomy patients need radiation.

Radiation therapy kills cells that are growing. In a normal breast, only a few cells are actually growing at any one time; a cancer consists of cells that are growing all the time. Radiation therapy, therefore, has its greatest effects on cancer, although it inevitably causes some damage to other tissues. This damage can result in slight scarring of the breast.

HOW IS RADIATION THERAPY DONE?

You will probably be asked to come to the outpatient clinic each weekday for five to seven weeks to have radiation treatments. It takes only a few minutes each time and is completely painless, a bit like having an X-ray.

You do not need to worry that it will make you radioactive. Before you are given the first dose, a semi permanent dye is used on your skin to mark the area to be treated. This ensures that whoever is giving the treatment can place you in exactly the same position each time. You will be asked to keep absolutely still during therapy.

After a few days of radiation therapy, your skin may look red and feel a bit sore, as if you had spent too long in the sun. Toward the end of treatment, you may also experience some blistering of the skin. Since wetting the skin can make it sore, some radiation therapists prefer patients to keep the treated areas dry and just apply creams. Others do not object to getting the area wet. Your radiation therapist will determine what is best for you. You should protect the treated area from the sun.

Today, there are very few side effects from radiation therapy. It does not make your hair fall out or make you nauseated, although toward the end of the treatment you can feel tired. Some patients who receive radiation to the breast get a cough because some of the radiation penetrates the part of the lung immediately under the breast. This can cause scarring of the lung, which causes irritation and results in a cough or, occasionally, shortness of breath. If you experience these problems, you should report them to your own doctor since there are specific treatments for these symptoms.

FOLLOW-UP APPOINTMENTS

If you have had breast-conserving surgery, you will probably have to go for a checkup every six months for several years. You should get mammograms of both breasts every year. If you have had a mastectomy, your checkups will probably be every six months for the first year and then annually, with mammograms of the remaining breast every year.

DRUG TREATMENTS

Drugs have an advantage over treatments such as surgery and radiation therapy because they reach all parts of the body. Drugs can act on cancer cells that have spread in such small numbers that they cannot be detected. As a result, drugs can prevent the recurrence of cancer for months or even years after treatment. If cancer is already widespread by the time it is first diagnosed, drugs may be the only practical way of treating it.

The drug treatment used for breast cancer falls into two main categories: hormones and chemotherapy.

HORMONES

Most breast cancer is affected by hormones and mainly by estrogen. The other natural hormones that affect breast cancer are progesterones. At low levels, progesterones do not seem to have much influence. When given in high doses, however, progesterones can make breast cancer shrink as effectively as any other hormonal manipulation, such as removing estrogen or using anti-estrogens (see pp.75–76).

It is possible to determine whether a tumor is sensitive to hormones by doing a chemical test on tumor specimens that are taken during the biopsy. Most breast cancers are estrogen-sensitive, so that the presence of estrogen increases the rate at which the cancer cells multiply. There is a tendency, however, for younger women to have a slightly higher incidence of hormone-insensitive cancers. After menopause, women tend to have a high incidence of hormone-sensitive cancers.

● **Estrogen-sensitive tumors** In postmenopausal women, about two out of three have estrogen-sensitive tumors; the proportion is closer to one-half for pre-menopausal women. These hormone-sensitive cancer cells have receptors on their surface that react to estrogen, causing the cells to multiply more quickly.

Tamoxifen is a drug that works by blocking the effects of estrogen on the tumor. In some patients this results in tumor destruction; in others it prevents further growth of the tumor. Either of these effects can be of great benefit in controlling the disease and eliminating the symptoms of the cancer. The effect of tamoxifen may last for many months or years in certain patients, although it is impossible to predict just how long the effect will last.

The only really serious side effect is that tamoxifen can double the incidence of endometrial cancer in the lining of the womb. There is no doubt that this risk has been overemphasized in the media, and the actual risk is very low. If tamoxifen is taken for no more than five years, the risk of developing endometrial cancer is extremely low.

Most of the evidence suggests that, for protection against breast cancer, the optimum length of time to take tamoxifen is probably 5 years.

OTHER DRUGS

A new class of drugs for treating breast cancer, called aromatase inhibitors, has become available within the last few years and is proving to be beneficial. They are used in women who are postmenopausal, and they act by blocking the production of estrogen, which is still made in considerable quantities in these women. In blocking the production of estrogen, they deprive breast cancer cells of estrogen, which acts as a stimulant to the cancer cells. This is the only way in which their action is similar to the effect of tamoxifen. Aromatase inhibitors can work after tamoxifen has failed to control tumors. They are well tolerated and are being tested as alternatives to tamoxifen in the treatment of the early stages of the disease.

Progesterones are also used to treat breast cancer in a large number of patients. They are often used after initial therapy with tamoxifen or one of the new aromatase inhibitors has failed. The way in which progesterone actually works is complex and poorly understood, but the drugs do have a very good, long-standing track record for controlling the disease.

The main reasons for choosing tamoxifen or aromatase inhibitors ahead of the progesterones are the side effects. These side effects are mild or minimal with tamoxifen and aromatase inhibitors, but they can be more troublesome with the high-dose progesterones, in particular the weight gain. A glance at the side effects of drug treatments (opposite) gives some insight into the most common side effects seen with hormone therapy and which drugs are especially associated with particular side effects.

CHEMOTHERAPY

Chemotherapy consists of a combination of anticancer drugs, often two or three at a time. These drugs are intended primarily to identify and kill cells that are actively growing and dividing. Unfortunately, anticancer drugs are not able to recognize cancer cells specifically, and, consequently, they kill other actively dividing cells such as cells of the blood, bone marrow,

Side Effects of Hormonal Treatments

Unfortunately, many hormonal treatments have unpleasant side effects. The most common ones are listed below. However, a patient may not necessarily suffer from any or all of the side effects.

THERAPY	SIDE EFFECTS
Ovarian Ablation (Surgical Removal of Ovaries)	Menopausal hot flashes and sweats, joint stiffness, decreased sex drive, and vaginal dryness.
Tamoxifen	The effects listed above plus weight gain, transient nausea, effects on the eyes, endometrial cancer risk, and blood clots.
Specific Aromatase Inhibitors	As for ovarian ablation, plus nausea.
Progesterone	Increase in appetite, weight gain, vaginal bleeding, and blood clots.
Specific Antiestrogens	No menopausal hot flashes or sweating.

and hair. The bone marrow is an extremely important tissue in the body because it produces the blood cells and the cells of the immune system that fight infection. Drugs that destroy these cells produce complications such as anemia, tendency to infection, and, rarely, problems with blood clotting that result in a tendency to bleed after minor injury.

The main effect on the blood, however, is on the white cells, which are part of our defense against infection. Because of their rapid turnover, white blood cells are particularly sensitive to the damage caused by toxic chemotherapy drugs.

The art and science behind successful cancer chemotherapy lie in deciding on the right combination of drugs to use. Drugs are chosen to cause minimal damage to the blood and maximum damage to the cancer cells.

Sometimes chemotherapy is administered prior to surgery in order to shrink the tumor, so that the surgeon can leave more of the breast undamaged by the operation.

Cancer chemotherapy is usually given through an intravenous drip into your arm. Treatments vary, but each session usually takes between one and three hours, is repeated every three weeks, and can be done on an outpatient basis. Some patients may well be frightened by the prospect of having chemotherapy because they have heard that there are unpleasant side effects, such as nausea, vomiting, and hair loss. In actual fact, not everyone experiences all or even any of these problems. Antinausea medicines given with the chemotherapy work very well. Sedatives and/or antinausea drugs can be given through an intravenous drip if necessary.

One of the lesser-known side effects of chemotherapy is premature menopause. This is particularly likely to occur in women in their late 30s and 40s. Even younger patients can experience a temporary cessation of their

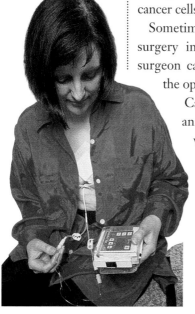

CANCER-KILLING DRUGS
This chemotherapy pump is worn by the patient and allows a measured dose of anticancer drugs to be administered continuously into a vein near the shoulder.

menstrual periods due to the effects of chemotherapy on hormone production by the ovaries. In younger patients, menstrual periods typically return some time after the course of chemotherapy is completed, but natural menopause may occur several years early.

Except in the youngest patients, chemotherapy is likely to impair fertility. To preserve the possibility of having a family after they have been treated for breast cancer, some women may want to attempt egg storage before having chemotherapy. The most reliable means of accomplishing this is to visit a specialist in infertility medicine with your partner and arrange for the storage of your fertilized eggs, known as in vitro fertilization, or IVF. Researchers are now looking into the possibility of storing unfertilized eggs, but at the moment that is an unproven and unreliable technique.

Chemotherapy does not impair a woman's fertility in every case. It is therefore advisable to avoid becoming pregnant by using a barrier method of contraception such as a condom because contraceptive pills can have an adverse effect on the breast cancer.

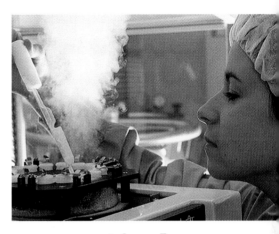

STORING EGGS
Placing fertilized eggs in storage may be recommended for women who need chemotherapy treatment, which can cause infertility.

▪ HORMONE REPLACEMENT THERAPY ▪

Chemotherapy and hormone therapy can produce menopausal symptoms and may artificially induce permanent menopause. Many patients ask whether it is possible just to use hormone replacement therapy (HRT) to relieve the unpleasant symptoms of menopause. Most often, the advice is not to take hormone replacements until alternatives have been tried, although no one is entirely certain if hormone replacement therapy adversely affects breast cancer or not. The problem is that hormone replacement therapy is made up of low doses of estrogen, which, in theory, can stimulate some forms of breast cancer to grow again. Trials are being conducted to find out whether hormone replace therapy can be safely used, but the results of this research will not be available for several years. There are other ways of alleviating menopausal symptoms that are caused by anticancer treatments. These may sometimes involve using drugs, such as low-dose progesterones. In some cases, lifestyle changes, such as wearing loose-fitting clothes that are made of natural rather than synthetic fibers, can be helpful in decreasing discomfort by reducing sweating.

COMPLEMENTARY MEDICINE

Most doctors are concerned about the idea of patients who have breast cancer opting solely for treatment through alternative forms of medicine because their disease is so eminently sensitive to conventional treatment. Nevertheless, many people find great comfort in taking a hand in the control of their condition by visiting herbalists or other practitioners.

The commonsense approach is to discuss this openly and honestly with your primary care physician. He or she is unlikely to object, provided that you do not choose complementary medicine in place of conventional medical treatment.

— WHEN A CURE IS NOT POSSIBLE —

Despite the best efforts of medical and surgical teams, some women with breast cancer will go on to develop advanced disease that cannot be cured. Even when this does happen, however, there is still an enormous amount that can be done to help both the woman and her family.

It is nearly always possible to control symptoms such as pain and nausea, and palliative care teams have the necessary expertise. In this context, the palliative care team can advise either the patient's doctor or the hospital oncology department about the optimum use of analgesics and drugs that combat nausea and diarrhea, as well as how to maximize the patient's appetite, which can often be poor as a result of the illness or the treatment. The main aim in this instance is to give the patient the best possible quality of life, with minimum symptoms of the disease and minimum side effects of treatment.

For information about organizations that can provide information and support, see pages 86–87.

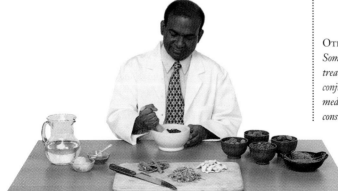

OTHER TREATMENTS
Some forms of complementary treatment may be used in conjunction with conventional medicine, but be sure to consult your doctor.

KEY POINTS

- Synthetic hormones are very effective drugs for treating hormone-sensitive breast cancer.
- Chemotherapy doses and schedules are optimized to give the best anticancer effect while causing the least damage to normal tissues.
- Palliative treatment of breast cancer is often done in conjunction with an expert care team whose aim is to improve the patient's quality of life.

Personal reactions

Any breast problem, even one that is minor, is likely to affect a woman psychologically and emotionally as well as physically. Many women are sensitive about the shape and size of their breasts and how they relate to their sexuality.

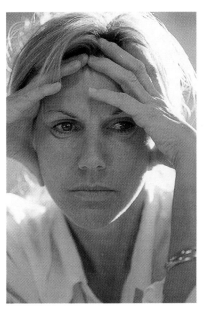

Both men and women perceive breasts in a sexual way, and a woman may be concerned about her partner's likely reaction as well as her own to any breast problem.

From her own perspective, anything that is wrong with her breasts may have a damaging effect on her self-image and therefore takes on an importance far beyond its significance in pure health terms. Of course, no two women will react in exactly the same way, and your reaction to a breast problem is unique. Still, knowing that these kinds of concerns are normal may help you keep them in proportion.

Doctors and nurses who treat women with all kinds of breast problems are well aware of the psychological aspects of breast disease. Usually, they ask about your emotional reactions and whether you have concerns you would like to discuss. It really is worth taking this opportunity to bring up anything that is on your

THE EMOTIONAL RESPONSE
The psychological impact of breast cancer can be devastating. The loss of a breast can be a major blow to a woman's self-esteem.

mind. Some people find this difficult, perhaps feeling that nothing can be done to help or that they would be wasting the professionals' time. This is not the case, and keeping your concerns to yourself is likely to do more harm than good in the long run.

You should be offered support and advice by the doctors and nurses involved in your care. There are also numerous support groups that can offer something more for those who want it. In particular, a lot of help is available for women who have breast cancer and their families. Support groups can provide the opportunity to meet and talk to others in a similar situation. Usually the support contact had breast cancer that was treated successfully and has had some training in helping other people cope. Details can be found in the Useful addresses section (see pp.86–87).

When a family member or close friend has a serious condition such as breast cancer, it can be difficult to

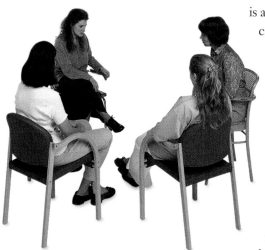

GETTING SUPPORT
Self-help groups can prove to be a valuable source of emotional support, as can your specialized care team.

express your own worries or seek emotional support for yourself. Many relatives believe that they must not compete with the patient's need for help even though they may have as many or more concerns. There are now many groups to help relatives cope with breast cancer.

KEY POINTS

- Breast conditions can often affect women psychologically and emotionally.
- Do not keep your concerns to yourself; instead, share them with your caregivers and family.
- Support should be available from your doctors and nurses and is also available from self-help groups.

Useful addresses

Support groups

If you would like to talk to someone who has been through similar experiences, trained volunteers can be contacted through organizations such as Y-ME or local self-help groups. The following national associations provide emotional support and practical help for women with breast cancer and their friends and relatives.

American Cancer Society

Online: www.cancer.org
1599 Clifton Road
Atlanta, GA 30329
Tel: (800) 227-2345
Tel: (404) 320-3333

American Society of Breast Disorders

Online: www.asbd.com
PO Box 140186
Dallas, TX 75214
Tel: (214) 368-6836

Cancer Care, Inc.

Online: www.cancercare.org
1180 Avenue of the Americas
New York, NY 10036
Tel: (800) 813-HOPE

National Alliance of Breast Cancer Organizations (NABCO)

Online: www.mabco.org
9 East 37th Street, 10th floor
New York, NY 10016
Tel: (212) 889-0606
Fax: (212) 689-1213

National Cancer Institute

Online: www.rex.nci.nih.gov
Building 31, Room 10A07
31 Center Drive MSC 2580
Bethesda, MD 20892
Tel: (800) 422-6237
Tel: (301) 496-5583

National Coalition for Cancer Survivorship

Online: www.cansearch.org
1010 Wayne Avenue, Suite 550
Silver Spring, MD 20910
Tel: (301) 650-9127

National Lymphedema Network and Hotline

Online: www.lymphnet.org
2211 Post Street, Suite 404
San Francisco, CA 94115
Tel: (800) 541-3259

National Women's Health Network
Online: www.womenshealthnetwork.org
1325 G Street, NW
Washington, DC 20005
Tel: (202) 347-1140

Revlon/UCLA Breast Center
Online:
www.med.ucla.edu/womens/revlon.htm
200 UCLA Medical Plaza, Suite B265
Los Angeles, CA 90095
Tel: (800) 825-2144

Strang Cancer Prevention Center
Online: www.strang.org
428 East 72nd Street
New York, NY 10021
Tel: (800) 521-9356
Tel: (212) 794-4900

The Susan G. Komen Breast Cancer Foundation National Headquarters
Online: www.komen.org
5005 LBJ Freeway, Suite 370
Dallas, TX 75244
Tel: (800) IM-AWARE
Tel: (972) 233-0351

The Wellness Community
10921 Reed Hartman Highway,
Suite 215
Cincinnati, OH 45242
Tel: (888) 793-WELL

Y-ME National Breast Cancer Organization
Online: www.y-me.org
212 West Van Buren
Chicago, IL 60607
Tel: (800) 221-2141
Tel: (312) 294-8513

Notes

Notes

Notes

Notes

Notes

Index

Acknowledgments

PUBLISHER'S ACKNOWLEDGMENTS

Dorling Kindersley Publishing, Inc. would like to thank the following for their help and participation in this project:

Managing Editor Stephanie Jackson; **Managing Art Editor** Nigel Duffield; **Editorial** Mary Lindsay, Irene Pavitt, Jennifer Quasha, Ashley Ren, Design Revolution; **Design** Sarah Hall, Design Revolution, Chris Walker; **Production** Michelle Thomas, Elizabeth Cherry.

Consultancy Dr. Tony Smith, Dr. Sue Davidson; **Indexing** Indexing Specialists, Hove; **Administration** Christopher Gordon.

Illustrations (p.11, p.17, p.24) Neal Johnson, (p.9, p.22, p.70, p.73) ©Philip Wilson, (p.60) Fiona Roberts.

Picture research Angela Anderson; **Picture Librarian** Charlotte Oster.

PICTURE CREDITS

The publisher would like to thank the following for their kind permission to reproduce their photographs. Every effort has been made to trace the copyright holders. Dorling Kindersley apologizes for any unintentional omissions and would be pleased, in any such cases, to add an acknowledgment in future editions.

APM Studio p.32, p.33
National Medical Slide Bank p.28, p.43, p.47, p.48;
Science Photo Library p.3, p.15 (King's College School of Medicine), p.14 (Chris Priest), p.20 (Hattie Young), p.26 (King's College School of Medicine), p.30 (Dr. P. Marazzi), p.46 (Dr. P. Marazzi), p.50 (Breast Screening Unit, King's College Hospital), p.53 (Chris Bjornberg), p.61 (Nancy Kedersha), p.63 (BSIP, Laurent H. Americain), p.65 (BSIP Boucharlat), p.66 (King's College School of Medicine), p.78 (James King-Holmes), p.79 (Hank Morgan), p.83 (BSIP Chassenet); **Telegraph Colour Library** p.19 (R. Chapple); **Tony Stone Images** p.16 (Ben Edwards).